ERROR: Programmer Burnout

404 Joy Not Found

```
/*****
The missing How-to manual for computer programmers (and managers) who struggle
with the Invisible Beast of workplace misery.  How to spot the signs, regain
productivity AND also have a life.

@params: Attention, consideration, willingness to make some subtle changes
@output: Your Life
@author: Burt N. Crispy
******/
```

Table of Contents

How to Read This Book

or, Find your own way

Start anywhere, and <u>read it several times</u>.

This book is meant for computer programmers, it's really slanted for them, but it applies to anyone who has been experiencing unhappiness in the workplace.

This book is not merely theoretical. If you obtained it then you are probably in crisis (even if you are not yet aware of it) and you need to take strategic action now to change your situation for the better. It's full of practical tips, (mostly just two major ones). I will urge you over and over to <u>actually go and do</u> what I recommend, like, right away, right now. None of this book will do anything for you unless you give it a try in your real life. So, be prepared to put down the book at a moment's notice and follow through on my recommendations, quickly, before you can over-think about it and miss the potential benefits. Don't worry, you will always get another chance to act.

Learn from my bad life story. Apply wisdom and change your behaviors before the problem gets really bad.

Forward

OK, first things first. Workplace Burnout can be very serious. There's no easy way to say this so I'll jump right into the deep end … If you're thinking of jumping off a bridge or blowing your brains out, <u>Don't do it!</u> Things will get better, they really will. I know it doesn't seem like it now but they will improve, you can be happy again, and there are actually people out there who want to be your friend, even if only a little and from a distance. If you are thinking about ending it at all, if you yearn for the peace of death, go straight to your doctor's office and quietly inform the receptionist that you need to see the doctor right away and it's very *very* important, now (when she asks you "what it's about", say "it's private"). Don't leave the waiting room, stay. A doctor can hear you out and give you immediate relief in the form of an anti-depressant. I know, it's cheating, and it's not a long-term solution, but it will reduce your pain and clear your head, which is what you need for the time being. Ask the doctor to write you a note saying you can't work for medical reasons, it might come in handy later. You can also phone a suicide hotline any time of the day or night. They'll talk you down off the ledge, which is a beautiful service they provide, for free. You're not alone. Lots of people have been stuck in that hopeless place and lived to tell about it. I did. You're going to be OK. You've got this.

Next, don't quit your job, not just yet. You might decide to quit later, but for now just reduce your hours or responsibilities, and play it cool until your brain is back to normal. Don't make any final decisions yet.

Do <u>not</u> take revenge. That kind of thing always blows back at you.

Next, it's okay to take a "medical stress leave", it is a perfectly fine and normal thing. You're not the first one to do so. Other people are burning out all over the place, left and right. It's a big problem in our society right now all over the industrialized world. You won't get fired for asking for a stress leave, although your boss will probably hate the idea, he can't stop you, and he may even be sympathetic (and if he fires you then at least you know you were actually working for an unsympathetic asshole, and now you're free!). If your doctor gives you a note then you could even apply for unemployment benefits. If you live in a truly civilized country like Sweden, you can even get a year off and skills retraining, supported by the taxpayer. But don't worry about money, at this point you need to take care of yourself, first priority.

You need to get your heart and brain back to normal... now. I'll do my best to show you how to do that in the shortest time possible, then show you how to back that up with strong long-term strategies.

A Brief History of How I Went Up In Flames,

or "Do I smell smoke? Oh, it's just my brain melting down"

By now you must have realized that I burnt out, and now I'm writing a book about it, so it must have been pretty bad. It's true, I worked and worked on a project that I wasn't really passionate about because it was available, it was a good technical match, the boss had money, and most importantly *I was responsible for supporting my family, and I was happy to take on that burden*. (To clarify: Supporting my family is a good thing which I am more than happy to do, but I sacrificed my well-being too much for the job, and it nearly broke me.) I hoped to make a success of the company so that I could further my career and keep my family fed. I aimed to put in 110%, to be a "star employee". At first it was good, I worked alone and had many early successes, but then there was some friction, like the boss kept insisting on very short deadlines for huge tasks, which I allowed. I just stayed up late and did the deed. Delayed payments, I allowed. Phone calls on weekends, I allowed. Work through holidays, I allowed. Yelling over the phone, I allowed. Wage raise refused, I allowed. Request to bring on more programmers refused, I allowed.

Are you seeing a pattern here? I allowed Bad Management. There was friction, and it started to cause heat and smoke in my human meat body suit. I began to complain to my wife and kid. They told me to stand up for myself but I didn't want to jeopardize the job. It went on and on, it was almost hypnotic, I was tired and disheartened but just shook it off with coffee and resolve. The boss gave me the constant impression that he was deep into debt and had no money for me, which was not true, but I allowed. I kept making excuses for him, I thought he and I were scrappy entrepreneurs out to make a success, together as a "team". The business had a big potential upside. He promised that when the program made money that he would "take care" of me, I allowed ....

Well, anyway, it went on for years, him withholding budget and benefits and me busting my chops, but at least he was paying me regularly now. We brought on new super-talented programmers. Actually, I found them, I hired them, trained them, and managed them. I asked for a manager's wage but was refused, which I allowed. Work, work, train train, hire hire, manage manage, coffee coffee. Getting more and more tired. No holidays. Now we were making money and I actually got a wage increase. Yay! I could hire helpers as long as they're cheap.

Here's a good one: I'm Canadian so I can't take American holidays. I can't take Canadian holidays because it's an American company. I don't get employee benefits because I'm a consultant. I don't get a high pay because I'm "one of the family" (but not really). Which I allowed. At this point smoke began coming out of my ears.

OK. You're numb by now. You must think I'm a big whiner, and you're right, I was reduced to a pathetic whiner, a Depressed Loser. "Just quit" you would say, but I was already deep into the burnout trap and I didn't know it. The signs were there but I just couldn't see them. I started taking Ritalin and Starbucks to power through deadlines. I was running on stimulants and my frontal brain was slowly shutting down from stress. I sent out resumes a few times but never got a response because I was so tired I couldn't focus on a job search. My resume was out of date, I didn't have time to catch up with new technologies, I was starting to hate programming (which I formerly loved), my productivity was suffering, and I had allowed so many insults that my self-worth was getting seriously eroded. In hindsight, I should have quit at this point, but I bought the idea that more "hard work" was all I needed to finally get recognized and rewarded. Man, was I wrong....

Flash forward to year 5... There are forty people in the company. Communication is horrible between the three primary department heads, there is absolutely no synergy. My self-esteem is in the shit can. I had to give up Ritalin because it gave me anger flares. I'm drinking gin in the evenings in an effort to self-soothe. My boss has continuously ignored my every request, but denies it, telling me "I gave you everything you ever asked for". I allow it. I have ingeniously patched together a working system with a skeleton crew of inexpensive foreign programmers, who I can barely manage anymore because I've had to take on every task that can't be done by them, so I have no time to write specifications and to manage them, they are wandering loose. We are on a Death March, we can't even keep up with maintenance. Customer demands and complaints are just forwarded directly to me from front desk, and I'm expected to customize a solution and have it in production the same day – which I'm able to do somehow, by the grace of the Computer Gods, but, not always. There is one low-talent programmer I hired in the early stages who has decided he will become my enemy and get rid of me by slandering me, let's call him Shylock. Shylock moves to the same neighborhood as my boss and becomes a sycophant. He is made into a department head. Shylock likes to yell at me in meetings, blaming me for every problem, hoping the boss will think he's real "Executive Material". My request to have him reprimanded is ignored due to nepotism. I allow it. There is another programmer I hired later on who has decided to create his own little empire of secret freelancers, and convinced the boss that he should have my job by bragging about massive untrue claims and promises, let's call him (who's a famous mutineer?) Lieutenant Fletcher. (from *Mutiny On The Bounty*) Well, they got together and kicked my nuts real hard one day, and replaced me with the mutinous Lt. Fletcher. Shylock wrote me a slimy "nice" private message to gloat over my loss. My boss just let it happen, because he didn't give a fuck about me, and I think he liked to watch people fight for his own entertainment.

And that's when it happened. Boom! I "burned out". Years of frustration and fear came crashing in. Panic attacks erupted day and night. The anxiety attached itself to my neck and shoulder. I got a searing pain in my upper back, as if I had been stabbed in the back (metaphoric, eh?). I became allergic to … everything. My immune system tanked. My mind was filled with constant dialogs of hatred and outrage. I couldn't sleep worth a damn. That's when I went to the doctor, she gave me anti-suicide pills and she wrote me a note recommending a six month leave.

I took off two months and went to the beach, unpaid of course, my boss insisted it was all my fault ... my mind was still boiling, and my body was in so much pain I only enjoyed the last week or so. I returned to work but all the same bullshit was there waiting for me, except that now Lt. Fletcher was to be my new boss. He immediately began a subtle harassment campaign. Ugh.

I struggled on for another month, but couldn't focus at all, so I finally <u>quit</u>, and my request for a severance package was (you guessed it) refused. I allowed it. My wife and I celebrated that evening anyway. I slept that night like a baby. The next day I began to feel really really good. I could literally feel my brain turn on again and my soul return to my body, after months of distraction and pain.

So that's my brief story. What went wrong here? Well, as it turns out, a lot, but it wasn't all my fault, though some of it was my fault, and I could have done many things earlier if I just had the right guidance. This little book is an attempt to help people before it gets Bad. If you let it go on for too long, you will get a clinical depression, and that will *seriously fuck up your Joi de Vivre*. Don't follow my bad example, instead follow my good advice. But first, let's have a look at the Beast...

The Ugly Signs of Creeping Burnout,
or "Why am I so dumb? I didn't used to be dumb."

It's insidious, this slow choking of your soul. You don't see it coming. You just want to do a good job, you want to be recognized as a capable, competent person. You do your best, not every day, but you do as much as you can. You deserve to be treated well, but the insults are relentless, the shit keeps getting delivered on a conveyor belt, day after day. Nobody recognizes your accomplishments, they just give you more work. Slowly the resentment builds, the cortisol and adrenalin are released into your system every time you have a disgruntled thought. Squirt. Your body is now ready to fight or flee every minor threat, but there's nothing to fight, nowhere to run. You're stuck. The stress hormones are just left hovering around in your body and brain. After a little while they clear and you go back to work. That night you have a bad dream. No biggie.

When you wake up in the morning you're feeling a little more tired than normal so you buy a caffeinated beverage, which really gets you zooming along. It's not great for your brain function but at least you have the energy to get into the zone and get ahead of that deadline. You feel Hopeful. You can go for a long time like this but it's a lie. The caffeine and adrenalin are messing with your sleep, as are the bad dreams stemming from the insults. Your productivity begins to decline and you get into trouble, your bosses yell at you, they threaten and intimidate you because they learned their management techniques from some old Neanderthal textbook meant for flogging factory workers.

Oh shit! Now the adrenalin is coursing through your veins like a river. You give your head a shake, renew your holy vows to the computer gods and to your beautiful little family who loves you and relies on your paycheck. You gird your loins, pick up your broadsword, smash a can of Jolt Cola and get back to work. Only, here's the problem ... your frontal brain has gone offline, and you are totally unaware of it.

What do I mean by "frontal brain"? I'm glad you asked. In all animals, the brain has three parts, old, middle, and new. The new smart part is in the front of the head that's close to the senses, the middle part is where your mammalian emotions are kept, and the old lizard part is in the back that's close to the spinal chord. The new part, or neocortex is responsible for all the smart bits like thought, memory, reasoning, strategy, curiosity, math, programming, you know, all the things you need to earn a paycheck as a computer specialist. When the animal gets stressed by an external threat then the old and mid brains takes over. The new brain shuts down because it's not needed when you're fighting a bear with a sharp stick. Your body needs all the energy in the heart, lungs, and muscles. You are immediately ready to jump high, scream loud, and hit hard. Stab! Stab! KILL!!!

So, there you are, sitting in front of your computer terminal, Monster Cola running green in your veins. You're panting a little, sweating, dry mouth, hyper-vigilant, giving attention to any change in your environment, irritable, tense. You start fantasizing about martial arts movies, with yourself as the hero, defeating your enemies with swords and fists ….. You are "working", but any objective measure would show that you're not at your best; productivity has dropped off significantly. You work late into the night, you get into a fight with your family. Your sleep is now officially 8 hours of restless crapola. This cycle continuously repeats itself over weeks, months, even years, sometimes it gets better, but your brain's set point has changed into <u>permanent stress mode</u>, a sort of twilight condition where you are always mildly unhappy, living a life of quiet desperation, and utterly unaware that you are eroding away in several areas, like health, self-esteem, ingenuity, relationships, planning, joy, hope. Your spouse now starts to accuse you of procrastination and emotional blankness. It's true, you're frozen in place. You are probably sick and grumpy more often these days.

Congratulations! (sarcasm) Your ancestors are all shaking their heads. Your angels are crying for you. Jesus' heart is bleeding for you. Your soul is shriveling and dying... You have been slowly and secretly pulled, step by step, into the <u>Burnout Trap</u>.   You're in a trap, bro. This is what misery looks like. It's "Samara". Like a traumatized soldier, you now have PTSD. You have a major depression. We need to get out of it. Please believe me, there *is* a way out! We got into it step by step, so that's how we need to get out of it.

OK, switch scenes. Remember back to long ago, when you were a happy programmer. You used to love playing around with ideas, creating beautiful machinery that seamlessly merged multiple technologies. Your soul was free, it belonged to you. You felt proud of your accomplishments and were curious to learn more. You felt hopeful for your future. This is where you deserve to be! Healthy, whole, creative, with a full sense of worth. Look at all these areas where you deserve to be satisfied: Delicious food and drink, good friends, a good sex life, interesting fun activities, comfortable living conditions, a nice family scene, a workplace where you are respected and treated well. You can have this, all of it, you truly deserve it, even if you are skeptical now. I know you might not believe me yet, but stay with me.

Trust me, I'm going to help you, in the short-term and in the long-term. For the short-term, I'm going to give you some tricks to stimulate your brain into thinking that it's happy.

The Main Cause of Burnout,

or "It's true. They are completely at fault! …. Bastards…"

<u>You have been sold a lie that an ordinary life, honest effort and normal responsibility is not good enough, when in fact it is.</u>

But first, hear me, and I swear I'll make this brief... There is a great and horrible *moral injury* in this suffering world. Life is frequently cruel and horrible. Some people and some companies are <u>Takers</u>, meaning, they don't give a shit about you or your kids or your little dog either. They want to suck everyone's life force to gather to themselves more money and attention. They will tell you anything they think you want to hear so that they can continue to exploit your talents and your precious time. "It makes sense to be paranoid when bastards really are out to get you!" You need to identify and protect yourself from such people and such businesses. Test their integrity. Examine their words and their actions to see if they line up. Realize the truth. In these cases, you really are being used, manipulated, you're being taken for a ride. Or, they are simply too immature to have any real kind of two-way relationship with you. Do not waste your time on fake people. Don't be the sucker at the poker table. Organize your exit plan, and get out before your body and mind pay the price.

The world can be quite evil in some ways. It may take you a lifetime to come to terms with it. Try not to become evil yourself, as that would be to truly lose the whole game. Do your best to avoid becoming a victim, though.

If you are a programmer manager or executive reading this then *listen up* … Intimidation and fear will make your programmers dumb, ruining your prime business asset which is their Power of Creative Genius. They are not factory workers or farm slaves. You cannot threaten them, threats will *never* produce works of genius faster and faster. Just the opposite. Your smartest people will leave you and go elsewhere, where they are respected. You need to totally rethink your strategy. If you want the flower of genius to bring you the great wealth that you crave then treat your programmers like you would your own child (assuming you're not a sociopath). Don't manipulate them but instead give them what they ask for and treat them right.

Y'all need to learn a new skill, called <u>Discrimination, or Discernment.</u> Actually, you already have it, so the skill you need is to *trust* it. Follow your gut feelings, don't doubt your deepest emotions. Align with people and companies that accord with your highest truth and that give you a sense of hope. Look for the promotion track

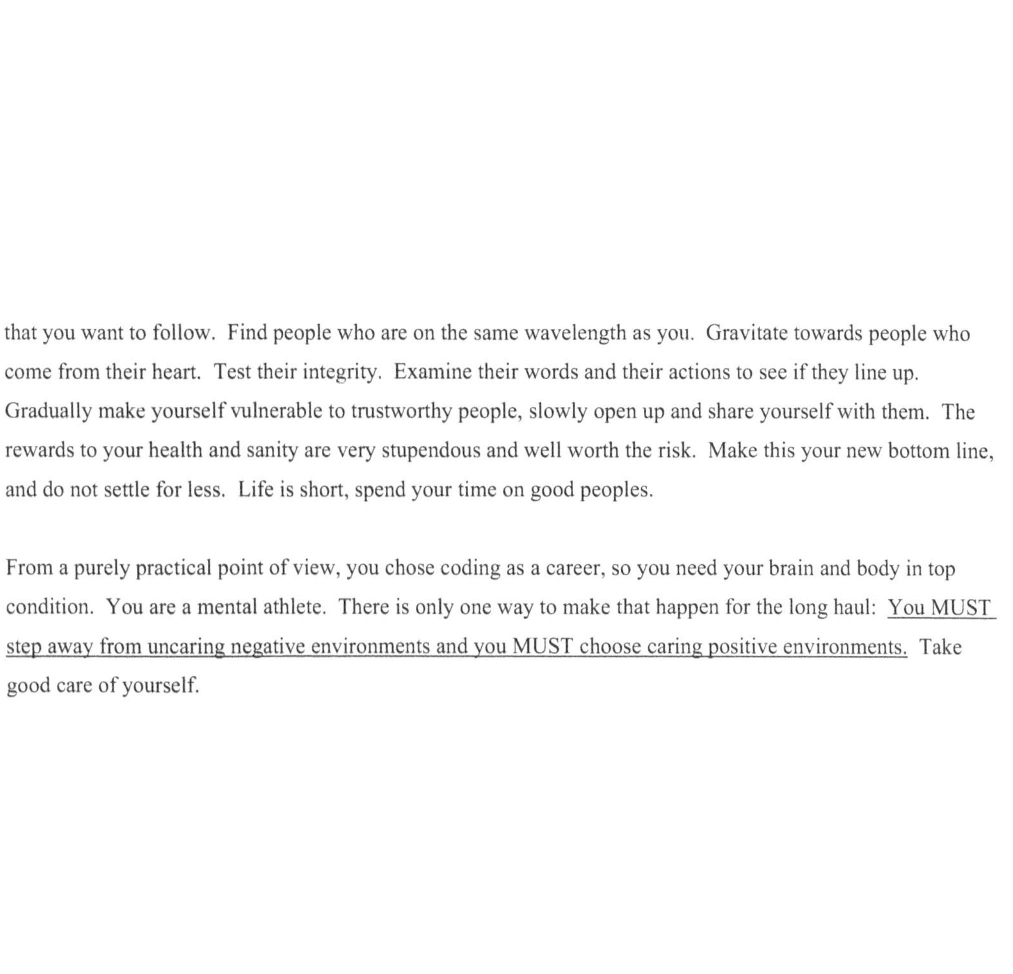

that you want to follow. Find people who are on the same wavelength as you. Gravitate towards people who come from their heart. Test their integrity. Examine their words and their actions to see if they line up. Gradually make yourself vulnerable to trustworthy people, slowly open up and share yourself with them. The rewards to your health and sanity are very stupendous and well worth the risk. Make this your new bottom line, and do not settle for less. Life is short, spend your time on good peoples.

From a purely practical point of view, you chose coding as a career, so you need your brain and body in top condition. You are a mental athlete. There is only one way to make that happen for the long haul: <u>You MUST step away from uncaring negative environments and you MUST choose caring positive environments.</u> Take good care of yourself.

The Very Easy Short-term Solution to Burnout Anxiety and Depression,

or "One weird trick that gives immediate, real relief"

OK, so now you know the seriousness of the problem, and have a good idea of how you got into a burnt out state. It will take a long time to fully heal and learn to trust again. But, for now you need to climb out of the stress hole quickly. You need first-aid. If you have found yourself deep into the burnout trap and are really feeling hopeless then don't forget to seek a mild anti-depressant drug treatment, you definitely need this crutch for a month or two, it will improve your recovery outcomes *greatly*. But more immediately, how do you turn off the panic attacks, fear, and anger, now? ... today? Is there an off switch? Yes. I've investigated a lot of techniques, and settled on this one. It's simple but very powerful if practiced in the right way:

I'm just going to put it out there, you're a smart person and you know that the human body can be conditioned, much like a computer can be programmed. How can you reprogram your human meat suit to calm down on command? It's actually very simple, and it's been known about for a very long time, throughout history. Ready? Here it is:

→ <u>**Breath regulation**</u> ←

I could try to give you a crash course here, and I will, but first go to Google and search for this term. You'll be amazed although probably not hugely surprised to find a million search results. Breath regulation is *A Thing*. The US Army teaches breath-work and yoga to soldiers to prevent and/or cure PTSD. Navy SEAL Teams use it to stay calm and focused during operations. The yogis were doing it in India five thousand years ago and still doing it today. Every religion has some kind of ritual for rhythmic breathing and body motions, like singing, chanting, bowing, circumambulating, mantras, prayers, call and answer, et cetera. Music calms our senses. Dancing makes us happy. Physiologists and doctors are very well aware of how regular, rhythmic breathing is crucial to health, just ask a surgeon, they monitor their patients' breathing patterns constantly and make life or death decisions based on what they observe. Athletes use it to give themselves peak performance. Executives pay thousands of dollars per day to learn these techniques in corporate wellness retreats.

So, you can use this for free. Air is free. *It will make you feel Free.* There are dozens of techniques you could use and they all work as long as they follow one crucial rule: <u>To reset your mind and body, the breath must follow a steady rhythm for about five minutes.</u> Now, I know that you may be overburdened and stressed out but

I need you to breath with me, right now. Trust me. Put down the book, close the door, turn off the phone, and breath nice and steady for five minutes or so. In. Out. Nice. And. Steady..... go on. Do it, and watch what happens.

(… later …)

Whoa. feeling pretty calm, eh? Keep up the rhythm while you keep reading. It feels good, doesn't it? You might feel little tingles and shivers as the heart gets nourishing oxygen and pumps red blood out to the peripheral nerves. The "fight and flight" reaction is being replaced by another reaction: "Rest and Digest" :) Breath. In. Out. Nice and steady. Keep it rolling, you're doing great. Your brain functionality is starting to turn on again. The feeling of fuzziness is beginning to fade away. The blood pH is normalizing. Your sense of curiosity is starting to return. Enzymes are releasing. Hormones are balancing. You are beginning to think of doing something nice, like going for a walk or phoning a friend.

Breath. In. Out. Nice and steady. Keep it rolling, you're doing great.

Pretty soon you're going to reset your brain back to a normal self-respecting mode. You can do rhythmic breathing anywhere, in the car, grocery shopping, waiting in lineups, walking, wherever you go. You have this amazing miraculous tool that you can carry with you anywhere, to use if you get stressed out. You are totally in control of it. <u>You can turn your neocortex back on again, and reset your body homeostasis back to normal, whenever and wherever you want to.</u>

Take some time to really appreciate this gift. Go for a walk alone and practice breathing in time. Go for a walk around the block... Go on.... Do it now …. This isn't a story book, this is your life. Go practice regulated breathing on a walk, now.

What To Do Now That You're Feeling Better

or "I have a life … really, I do!"

OK, you got your breathing turned back on again. Great! Now you need some rest. See if you can get yourself to sleep tonight. Take care of yourself, have a nice hot bath or shower. Do rhythmic breathing while you're bathing. Shut down your electronics and say good night to everyone. Turn down the lights and go into you room early. Prepare your bed. Take a little melatonin, or a warm glass of milk, or a sleepy-time tea. Do rhythmic breathing as you lie in bed falling asleep.

In the morning, as soon as you wake up, start rhythmic breathing again and (this is important!) get out of bed right away. Wash your face to wake up fully (cold water if you can stand it). Now you are well rested and ahead of the day's schedule. Take some time in the morning for yourself. Take care of yourself, whatever you need. Walk around the house in your housecoat. Hang out and have tea with your roomies. Pet the dog. Water your garden. Spend some quality time with your girlfriend. Whatever you need, it's your thing, do what you want to do. BUT! Don't engage with work yet!! Leave the electronics turned off. Set aside some time to <u>have a life</u> first thing in the morning, to set your day out on the right foot.

You know, when people are old and on their deathbeds, they never regret that they didn't do more work at the office, they regret they didn't do the things they love, like spend more time with their kids and dogs, or playing their favorite sports / music / hobbies, or having more sex. It really is the simple things in life that give it meaning. So go ahead and <u>seize those little moments of beauty</u>. Take mental photos of moments at the beach. Walk in the park at lunch time. Play guitar. Seduce your partner. Go have coffee with a friend. (And turn off that fucking smart phone when you're with other people! The constant interruptions are making you emotionally *dumb.*)

Find pathways of highest excitement. Your body is a finely tuned instrument, honed from millions of years of evolution. Your sense of excitement about persons, places, activities, and things is a message from deep in your limbic system / hippocampus / heart / guts / genitals / soul / God / universe / You-niverse. It is your navigation system, feeding you hints about what is sure to bring you the highest pleasure, satisfaction, and bliss. <u>TRUST your sense of highest excitement.</u> Follow your bliss. It is your best invisible friend beckoning you towards a happy future.

The Not-so Easy Long-term Cure for Burnout, Anxiety, and Depression
or "I need to fix some things, for real"

If you are deep into the burnout hole then it's possible that you literally can't think of a fun thing you would like to do. That is called "depression" my friend, and it might take a little while to pull out of it. Some researchers now believe that burnout is in fact a form of PTSD. Like an injured war veteran, you should get some therapy. <u>Book a therapy session right now</u>. While you're waiting, try a few days of serotonin-building activities. Serotonin is your body's natural happy drug, it gets released when you walk your dog or have great sex or any other blissful activity.

Serotonin-building bio-food:

1. Exercise until panting breath.
2. Probiotics once nightly
3. Foods containing complex carbohydrates or L-tryptophan
4. Vitamins B6, B12, and folate, as well as concentrates of saffron

[! warning: hard-hitting truth alert !]

This is gonna hurt. But ya, for sure, if you're burnt out then you need counseling, and here's why: You let people walk all over you and use you for a doormat. You didn't call them out when they were acting sketchy. You didn't confront the broken deals. You didn't push for what you needed. You mistrusted your gut instincts. You let them lie to you and you ate up their bullshit. You sacrificed more than you needed to. You overrode your common sense. You emotionally overreacted. You didn't follow your own moral guidelines. You let yourself down. Ouch.

This signifies something, not that you're a bad person or anything like that, but on the contrary, you feel things deeply, and you suffered a moral injury. But you did allow it to happen, you were complicit. Why? Now you need to dig deeper and find out if you also suffered emotionally as a child. Even one or two Adverse Childhood Events (or A.C.E.'s) can have a significant impact on the development of self-esteem. Even a passive injury like childhood emotional neglect can hurt you for life. It is probable that you are among the many millions of emotionally wounded people who now walk the world with a smile painted on their face and a little black hole in their hearts. You are not alone, it's kind of an epidemic, actually. That traumatic stress crap can get stuck in your brain and give you a subtle functional impairment, one that can really cause long-term trouble in your behaviors and customary reactions around career, friendships, and relationships. Long-term stress can also limit your brain's ability to grow new neurons (neurogenesis). It's worth having yourself checked out by a qualified therapist. If I'm wrong I will buy you a beer. But I'm not wrong. If you're burned out it's because you didn't defend yourself - you didn't think you were worth defending - *but you are so truly worthwhile, and lovable.* Go phone a therapist and set up an appointment. Start on that journey to self-esteem and learn how to take care of yourself in this crazy world. Go heal up that hole in your heart. Grieve that suppressed grief, don't be afraid. In all seriousness, go ahead and set it up now. You're life will change for the better, in ways you cannot yet imagine. You can be happy, you deserve it. When you find a therapist you know can help you then be prepared to work with them over the course of 10 sessions over a year, that's how long it takes to thoroughly decondition your childhood programming and learn all new positive self-esteem skills.

Take some time to study negotiation skills. You want to be able to feed your family or support your passion projects, which requires money. You need your genius mind to do that, therefore you must protect your greatest asset, your brain health. Learn how to be respectful and stand your ground. Learn how to conduct yourself in a meeting. Speak up for yourself. Stay tuned to truth. Take a negotiation class because you deserve to win a few, right?

If you still have a job, and the job you work at is not aligned to your higher values, makes you feel hopeless, or give you low self-esteem, then contact a good resume service and begin the task of searching for a better job. It might take a while if you need to update your skills. Or, who knows, the Universe is funny that way, it might show you the right job immediately. In any case, you will feel a sense of physical excitement when you see it, your emotions will respond. Trust your gut feelings. Don't ever take a job only because of money or ego. Start your job hunt early, check job boards daily or use a resume-blaster service, blast out lots of applications weekly, and start taking interviews. If you are truly excited in your soul, and you're sure you're a great fit for the company then go that extra mile to contact the owner of the company by phone or in person.

If you still have a job that you love (or think you could love again) but the people there are driving you fucking nuts, then you need to be very cautious now. You have to start your job search in secret now, before you burn out any further. You also need to start planning your exit strategies. AND, it's very important that you make amends with each person who is currently making you crazy. That will be difficult, but it is a fantastic opportunity to learn advanced communication skills. Who know?, you may even resolve your conflicts and renegotiate your position in the company to a point where you will be comfortable to work there again. Or, it could at least make the situation more bearable while you are looking for your new job.

If you are totally burnt out, hate everything about your job, and even the sight of source code makes you gag, be very very careful! You are at risk of dropping your entire career down the drain, wasting years of precious industry experience. Lots of people who burn out then go on to fully leave their industry! Don't become a statistic (unless you truly desire a new career). Don't let interpersonal issues and PTSD poison your mind against the things you used to love about your job. Get therapy, separate the career issues from the personal issues, you have to do this in therapy, it's not possible to do it on your own (you're smart but nobody can see their own blind spots). The residual resentment will linger in the background like a burning coal and burn down your career, sooner or later.

Let's talk about passion. Have you seen those job advertisements that want you to be "passionate about coding"? Passion seems to be the wrong word here. They're mistaken somehow. I mean, how many people get all juiced up and want to kiss their computer? You are passionate about your family, your lover, your motorcycle, your hobbies that fill you with joy. I think that I know what they mean though. They want employees who have intrinsic values that will be fulfilled by working for them. It's a smart question, in a way, because if you are passionately working to support your family, and if this company serves the public in a way that accords with your beliefs, or does something for society that you admire, then you will be *much* happier in the long run. But, managers need to inspire their employees, to give them something to look up to, they can't expect coders to come with pre-packaged passion! C'mon management, provide us with a compelling vision, a worthy goal, a plan that people can get excited about!

There are two types of motivations that drive every person: Intrinsic and Extrinsic. An intrinsic value is one that comes from inside of you, like putting on some music you really like, just for your own enjoyment. An extrinsic value is one that you look outside of yourself to fulfill, like paying your electric bill. Doing both will give you satisfaction, but in different ways. You need to pay attention to both and balance them out in your life. For our purposes here, it is important to know that slogging away for a company that you do not believe in will fatally erode your sense of well-being. Those who ignore their intrinsic needs are in danger of leading a miserable life. It's very important that you spend some time and effort discovering what it is that you are truly passionate about. What is it that gives you a sense of excitement and pleasure? Again, I say "follow your bliss", but of course you have to find it first. Make that a stated goal for yourself, to search out "What gives me happiness"? Discuss it with trusted friends and family. Take a weekend seminar. They may even encourage you to follow your dreams. You may doubt that you could make a career of your passions, but at least identify and do the things you love, and keep searching for a company that you would be proud to work for. Start small and build up. Life is short, enjoy it.

Career change may be coming on your horizon, maybe. If you find yourself daydreaming about it for hours a day, that's a pretty good clue. You have to really want it though, because it takes a ton of preparation and hard work, and there needs to be a proven market. But hey, if you can see yourself in those boots and it really makes you happy, then go for it! Try it out for free at first, just to gauge how it makes you feel. There are a ton of career change books out there, and career coaches. I recommend using both, *a lot!*

Your beliefs create your world. Firstly, your beliefs provide an internal chemical environment for the cells of your body. Secondly, your beliefs act like tuning forks which resonate with persons, places, and things in the outer world. Change your beliefs and you will change your perception of the world, which in turn will reveal to you those things which harmonize with them. This is the secret of life: watch your thoughts and change your thoughts to fear less and to accord with what you love.

Go get a piece of paper and a pen or pencil. Seriously, do it now, quickly, before you can overthink. This isn't a story-book, *it's your life, so take action*. OK, <u>write your belief words</u>. What are the first principles that you truly admire the most? Just, straight from the heart, quickly write the first word that pops into your head. For me it was "family", but for you it could be something else, maybe "freedom", whatever is your thing, I don't judge. Now keep at it, write down these power words as they rise up from your heart and mind. What do you most value and respect in life? What ideas and values make you feel proud? Spend some time on this, it's worth it because it's your soul, dude. Now take that paper and keep it somewhere you will see it every day. You could put it on your desk, on the wall, on the refrigerator. Just Do It. I won't tell you why, but I can *promise* that it will have a profound positive effect on you to see your Core Ideals written in front of your eyes every day.

The power of Intention. Once you actually <u>know</u> what you believe in, those beliefs will convert automatically into actions. Your sub-conscious mind is an expert at finding opportunity, it just needs the right program instructions. After you are clear on what you actually want in this world, repeat it to yourself, all sense of doubt and worthlessness will drop away, and be replaced by clear, present, conscious action. You will be working for yourself.

Stop trying so hard at things that don't matter to you, and start trying at things that do.

The Very Easy Solution to Burnout, Again,
it's worth repeating!

Follow one crucial rule: <u>To reset your mind and body, breathe intentionally for a brief period, the breath must follow a steady rhythm for about five minutes.</u>

Why am I going on and on about rhythmic breathing? Because it's fucking amazing, that's why.

Protect your greatest asset, your brain health. You are a brain athlete. Manage stress before it can ruin your brain functionality.

There is a growing pile of scientific evidence showing how mild regulated breathing positively affects the heart, lungs, brain, kidneys, liver, digestion, immune system, skin, bile ducts, you name any body part here. Nerve sheaths remyelinate. Hormones normalize. The immune system responds well. It makes you live longer! It reduces depression, anxiety, PTSD, infection, addiction, inflammation, erectile dysfunction, effective medicine dosage levels.... Et cetera.

Worth noting is breathing's effects on the heart. The heart beat becomes steady, which brings a lot of encouraging results, including a cohesive electric charge and harmonious magnetic field. Your heart produces about one or two watts of electric charge, which is propagated in waves throughout your entire nervous system, and emanates around the body in a toroid field, which others can sense. I have been told many times by friends and acquaintances after walking in the park while practicing intentional breathing that I "look great!". You might think it's just my experience, but I feel great and I feel like there's a ball of energy around me. Dogs come running up to me, people smile at me, friends hug me spontaneously, kids come over to me, people spark up conversations then say "thanks!" afterwards. That kind of feedback is great for the self-esteem. I gotta say it's a huge improvement from my overburdened, depressed gray-skinned self!

Religions have documented for centuries that when practiced for long periods of time, it brings the practitioner closer and closer to Enlightenment, or God-Realization. That's got to be a good thing, right? Living in a state of heightened awareness, presence, and bliss sounds like a desirable life outcome, or at least to me it does.

Rhythmic breathing is a dang Panacea!

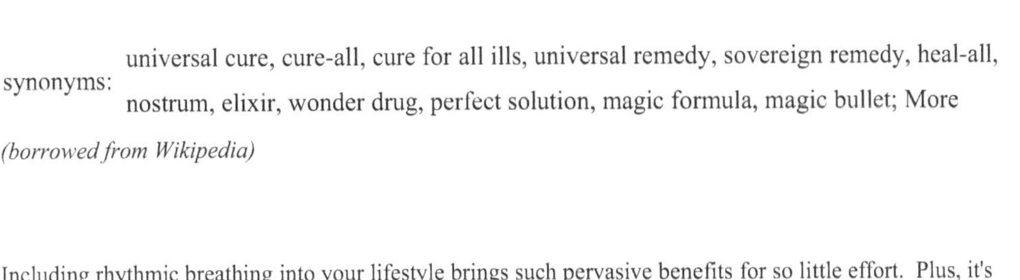

(borrowed from Wikipedia)

Including rhythmic breathing into your lifestyle brings such pervasive benefits for so little effort. Plus, it's immediately pleasurable … no down-side.

So seize your place in the world, take up your space, stand up straight and sovereign, proudly stand with your feet on the ground, open your heart, and breathe as much air as you want to. You belong here, and you have every right to ask for what you want, and to negotiate things to your satisfaction (respectfully).

Enjoy.

Extras

Extending your rhythmic breathing practice. These tricks will add extra sensory cues to help train your system to quickly exit "fight-or-flight" mode, and enter "rest-and-digest" mode. Once your brain is trained, it should take less than 20 minutes to calm yourself down and reach a balanced, focused state:

You could try to use a mantra in order to stabilize the breath, heart, and brain. It should be a short, repeatable phrase, preferably in a language you don't speak or understand, like Sanskrit for example. You say the mantra on the out-breath usually. You can say one syllable at a time, or the whole phrase, both techniques work because they do that crucial thing of regulating your breaths per minute. It adds a lot of stability to your practice, and drowns out your thoughts, which is especially helpful if you are in a thought-storm. Here are some common mantras, pick one and give it a try:

- **AHAM SOHAM** (Indian. Whisper "aham" on the in-breath, "soham" on the out-breath)
- **OM MANI PADME HUM** (Tibetan mantra of compassion)
- **HANA, TUL, SET, NET, TALSUT** (Korean, count your out-breath, one to five)
- **I AM THAT I AM** is a common English translation of the Hebrew phrase אֶהְיֶה אֲשֶׁר אֶהְיֶה, *'ehyeh 'ăšer 'ehyeh* – also "I am who I am", "I am what I am" or "I will be what I will be"
- **OM AH HUM** (Tibetan, focus attention on forehead, throat, and heart, respectively)
- [The name of your favorite God] (If you happen to be religious)

You could use a talisman stone or a rosary in order to cue your brain for the start, middle and end of a breathing session. Go to a spiritual gift shop and look at the stones, pick one that's appeals to you and is about the size of a dollar coin. Hold it in your hand when you do your rhythmic breath practice. Put it in your pocket and carry it around with you. Take it out and hold it when you are ready to start a session. It can be done anywhere and nobody will notice. Pretty soon your mind will come to associate holding the stone with a restful, coherent state. The same is true for a string of beads, a rosary or mala. You can also count off the beads one at a time as you count your breaths. I use my large mala at home. I like to walk while practicing but I don't always want people to see my mala, so I buy the ones you can wear as a bracelet that have an elastic string, you can slip it off any time and wrap it around your fingers, counting with the thumb. It conceals easily.

I recommend that you should tell only your closest people what you are doing. Don't talk about your breath practice or therapy to just anyone. Why? Because some dumbass is bound to say something stupid and put you off your game.   You are an a journey to regain your Soul here, so protect the secrecy of your practices like you would protect your cash stash – only tell those whom you trust implicitly and won't betray your confidence.

I should have warned you earlier that the anxiety you suffer from might begin to morph into anger or grief. This is a good thing, it means you're healing from subdued grief. Your mid-brain is waking up, coming online, and building new connections. Share your feelings with a close companion or counselor

Go for a walk every day *(and turn off your phone!)*. It resets your physiology, clears your head, and gives you a chance to daydream, which often gives birth to the best ideas.

Let's talk about neurogenesis, the development of new brain cells in the hippocampus (and possibly the cortex and hypothalamus). As programmers, we are mental athletes, <u>we absolutely need new brain cells</u>. There are several factors that increase and decrease it.

Increases Neurogenesis	**Decreases Neurogenesis**
Intermittent fasting	Junk food
Learning	Distress
Good sleep	Sleep deprivation
Exercise	Sedentary lifestyle
Omega 3 fatty acids	Saturated fatty foods
Socializing and human touch	Isolation and loneliness
Anti-depressants	Depression
Turmeric / curcumin	Chronic inflammation
Resveritrol, blueberries, red grapes, NMN	Alcohol
Youth	Aging

You could use this as a daily task-list for promoting neurogenesis in your own brain. You could also use it as part of an anti-aging regimen.

If you're feeling stressed out, you could try to stimulate your Vagus nerve. (No, it's not like that, dirty boy).
Splash cold water in your face, literally. The vagus nerve (or cranial nerve X) can be stimulated that way
because it has both sensory and motor function nerves which serve the face. It is the longest cranial nerve. It
runs all the way from the brain stem to part of the colon. The cold water stimulus gives your central nervous
system a nice friendly little shock, which is very good for it. You can also press your eyeballs when you dry
your face. And stick out your tongue and say "ah", plus gargle with cold water. Amazingly, that little cold
shock can lower your heart rate and kick-start your digestion. It's a great way to start your day and to refresh
yourself during breaks.

You might consider getting a dog, or just borrow one regularly PTSD therapy outcomes are often much better
with a "service dog". You should select a dog that's sweet and social, not too excitable, and who doesn't run
away if he gets off the leash.   Or, basically, any dog that you really like, and who really likes you.

Read up on the <u>Five Stages of Grief</u> by Elisabeth Kubler Ross & David Kessler
The five **stages**, denial, anger, bargaining, depression and acceptance are a part of the framework that makes up
our learning to live with the one we lost (or the boss/job we lost). They are tools to help us frame and identify
what we may be feeling. But they are not stops on some linear time-line in grief.

<u>Clinical depression</u> is marked by a depressed mood most of the day, sometimes particularly in the morning, and
a loss of interest in normal activities and <u>relationships</u> -- symptoms that are present every day for at least 2
weeks. In addition, according to the *DSM-5* -- a manual used to diagnose <u>mental health</u> conditions -- you may
have other symptoms with major depression. Those symptoms might include:

- <u>Fatigue</u> or loss of energy almost every day
- Feelings of worthlessness or guilt almost every day
- Impaired concentration, indecisiveness
- <u>Insomnia</u> or hypersomnia (excessive sleeping) almost every day
- Markedly diminished interest or pleasure in almost all activities nearly every day (called
  anhedonia, this symptom can be indicated by reports from significant others)
- Restlessness or feeling slowed down

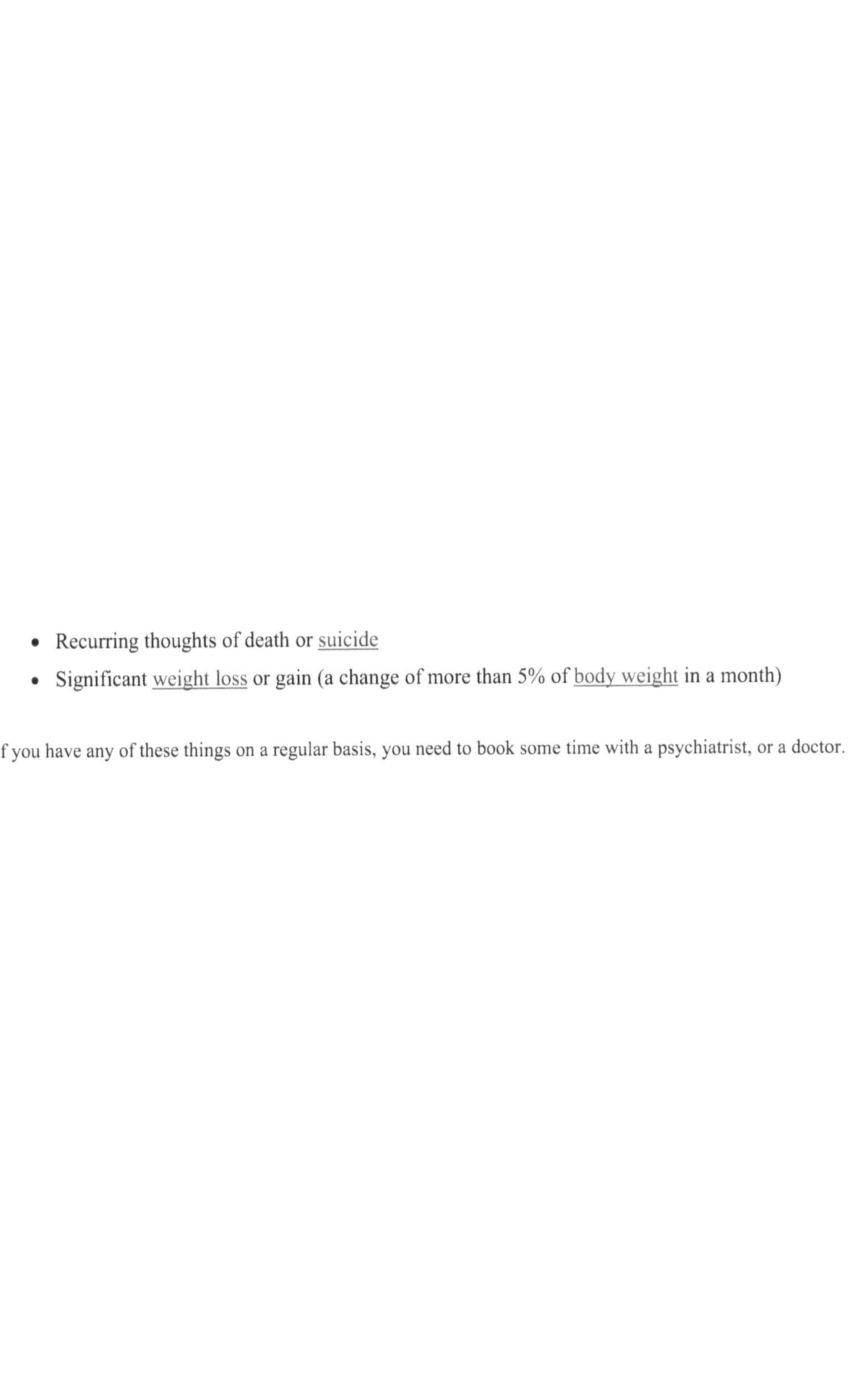

- Recurring thoughts of death or <u>suicide</u>
- Significant <u>weight loss</u> or gain (a change of more than 5% of <u>body weight</u> in a month)

If you have any of these things on a regular basis, you need to book some time with a psychiatrist, or a doctor.

Conclusion

OK, you finished the book. Good job! Now what? Go back to the beginning and read it again. Let the ideas really sink in. More importantly, do the activities recommended! Why?

It's your life, it's your happiness, so what are you going to do about it?

PS, Lend this book to your friends who are going through occupational depression and burnout. Please link to it in online discussions. If you borrowed this book, maybe you might want to buy your own copy? It's a lot of potential happiness for the cost of a coffee and a muffin. Just sayin' :)

Hmmm. Amazon says I need another 4 pages, so let's do a proper Conclusion section here:

Detailed Conclusion

- In the chapter <u>A Brief History of How I Went Up In Flames</u>, you saw my meltdown in extreme detail. It was a tailspin into Programmer-Hell.
    - An extreme pathological example of burnout
    - I have personal experience which qualifies me to give advice
    - A warning to change before things get ugly

- In the chapter <u>The Ugly Signs of Creeping Burnout, It's Root Causes</u>
    - Burnout comes on slowly
    - The signs are mainly physiological, not merely psychological.
    - It's a fight-or-flight syndrome. The smart parts of the brain shut down, blinding you to the progression of the syndrome, and reducing your productivity and planning
    - Family problems worsen, home life is affected
    - Sleep problems

- It feels like your "soul is dying"
- Burnout symptoms are virtually the same as Depression and PTSD

- In the chapter <u>The Causes of Burnout</u>, the source of the devil is made clear
  - Lack of self-protection within a hostile environment
  - You have been sold a lie that an ordinary life, honest effort and normal responsibility is not good enough, when in fact it is
  - Burnout is a moral injury. The work culture is toxic. You have been asked to behave in a way that is opposite to what you value and believe in.
  - Beware of the "Takers". You can identify them by the mismatch of words and actions, thereby revealing their true intentions.
  - Managers, you need to rethink your strategy. Intimidation and fear will make your programmers dumb, ruining your prime business asset which is their Power of Creative Genius.
  - You need to learn discernment. Learn to trust your gut.
  - You must learn to protect yourself, so that your brain can continue to work well!

- In the chapter <u>The Very Easy Short-term Solution to Burnout Anxiety and Depression,</u>
  - Burnout can take a long time to heal fully, but you need quick physical tricks to shut off the fight-or-flight syndrome as soon as possible.
  - The best trick is Breath Regulation, it has numerous benefits and no down-side. Just Do It.
  - Practice breathing every day in every situation -- it will have massive impact on your state of well-being.

- In the chapter <u>What To Do Now That You're Feeling Better</u>
  - Self care is vital for your recovery, and for quality of life.
    - Sleep
    - eat well
    - bathe
    - exercise
    - take plenty of time for your friends and family
    - get a dog
  - Seize those little moments of beauty, it's where life resides
  - Your sense of highest excitement, curiosity and bliss will lead you towards your best future.

- In the chapter <u>The Not-so-easy Long-term Cure for Burnout, Anxiety, and Depression</u>

  - You probably have a clinical depression. Come out of denial and get help. Set up therapy sessions.
  - Take action to build your serotonin.
  - Hard-hitting truth!: You acted like a door-mat and sacrificed your health. Why? You need to do a deep dive on this question, not to beat yourself up, but to find the core of your self-esteem, reclaim it, and nurture it.
  - Advice to take a negotiation course, learn how to stand up for yourself.
  - Strategize how to deal with your current job situation in the best practical way.
  - A discussion of passion, motivation, vision, love, beliefs, dreams, and goals
  - Take a weekend career-change seminar in order to discover what values are most important to you
  - Take action to write down your belief words on a sheet of paper, and post it where you can see it every day.
  - Stop trying so hard at things that don't matter to you, and start trying at things that do.

- In the chapter <u>The Very Easy Solution to Burnout, Again,</u>

  - To reset your mind and body, breathe intentionally for a brief period, the breath must follow a steady rhythm for about five minutes.
  - Get to know your Heart-Field. Learn to live in your heart.
  - **You belong here! Enjoy your life!**